MW00939945

MEMORIA

~~ORIGINAL EDITION~~

A Simple Book of Lists
to Exercise and Strengthen Your
Memory

CONNIE FINGER

Progressive learning is truly the Fountain of Youth and nothing will have you concede into aging more than believing you know it all.

Connie Finger

Dedicated to my mother, Maria, who passed away from Alzheimer's. To my brothers, family, friends and caregivers who, for the last 14 years of her life, gave of themselves to guide, care and govern her through a sickness that only declines. Attending to her condition made saints of them all.

Table of Contents

Preface

The requisite of memory is a lifelong essential for everyone. It is one of life's mental instruments needed to orchestrate a safe, productive, and well-lived existence while stockpiling a treasury of past remembrances. It is common to experience memory loss of some sort at various levels as we journey toward our senior years. Memory depletion sneaks up before one realizes it's a problem. We must all consider the value of our memories as we manage countless daily functions pertaining to ourselves and the world around us. Working out your memorization process (committing something to memory) will invigorate your memory system and help delay the approach of memory loss.

The goal of *Memoria*, is to help you achieve optimal memory efficiency by attempting to memorize as many of the lists provided. Every list is possible to memorize no matter how lengthy or difficult it may look. Compiled are 60 individual lists of assorted topics that are randomly catalogued. Each list features a wide range of difficulty to condition and fortify your memory. In the combat against memory loss, this book offers a simplistic exercise approach that is extremely user-friendly in processing your memory skills leading to dynamic results. Achieve a sense of triumph with every list your memory conquers. The more proficient you become in recalling the contents of each list, the stronger your power of retention will become. Curious users of this book are often inclined to strengthen their brain power by exploring and learning more about some of the topics introduced in *Memoria*.

AMAZE yourself and others with your mastery of *Memoria*!

How-To Instructions

There are none! Each individual has their own method of memorizing a list and everyone has a different retention level. Pick a list, any list, conquer it and go on to any other list. Feel like you hit a home run with every list you memorize. The object is to consistently exercise your memory at your own pace. Similar to repeatedly doing Tummy Crunches to strengthen your stomach muscles. Some lists are short & sweet and others are very challenging, in length and in content. Everyone has the potential of achieving total recall of any list in this book. Keep *Memoria* close at hand and establish a *Memoria* workout for the long run.

The contents of every list is current and factual according to the research. If a list ever becomes outdated, feel free to write in the necessary correction.

• • • • • •

Nations of the United Kingdom (4)

- England
- Scotland
- Wales
- Northern Ireland

Largest Rivers in the World (Top 5)

- Amazon River
- Congo River
- Chang Jiang (Yangtze) River
- Mekong River
- Yenisey River

Financial Markets (5)

- The Stock Market
- The Bond Market
- The Commodities Market
- Derivatives
- Forex Trading

Oceans (5)

- Pacific
- Atlantic
- Indian
- Arctic
- Southern (Antarctic)

• • • • • •

Principles of Reiki (5)

- Just for today: Do not anger
- Just for today: Do not worry
- Just for today: Be grateful
- Just for today: Work honestly
- Just for today: Be kind to yourself and others

Memoria   5

The Great Lakes of North America (5)

- Lake Huron
- Lake Ontario
- Lake Michigan
- Lake Erie
- Lake Superior

Types of Golf Clubs (6)

- Drivers
- Fairway Woods
- Hybrids
- Irons
- Wedges
- Putters

Space Shuttles, Flights, Orbits (6)

- Enterprise - 5 Flights - 0 Orbits
- Columbia - 28 Flights - 4,808 Orbits
- Challenger - 10 Flights - 995 Orbits
- Discovery - 39 Flights - 5,830 Orbits
- Atlantis - 33 Flights - 4,848 Orbits
- Endeavour - 25 Flights - 4,677 Orbits

● ● ● ● ● ● ●

Types of Triangles (7)

- Scalene
- Equilateral
- Isosceles
- Obtuse
- Acute
- Right Angled
- Oblique

Dwarfs in Disney's Snow White (7)

- Doc
- Grumpy
- Happy
- Sleepy
- Bashful
- Sneezy
- Dopey

● ● ● ● ● ● ● ● ●

States Served by the Colorado River (7)

- Wyoming
- Colorado
- Utah
- New Mexico
- Nevada
- Arizona
- California

Chakras (7)

- Crown Chakra/ Purple - "I understand"
- Third Eye Chakra/ Indigo - "I see"
- Throat Chakra/ Light Blue - "I talk"
- Heart Chakra/ Green - "I love"
- Solar Plexus Chakra/ Yellow - "I do"
- Sacral Chakra/ Orange - "I feel"
- Root Chakra/ Red - "I am"

● ● ● ● ● ● ● ● ●

Beer Types (8)

- Ale
- Cask Ale
- Kellerbier
- Lager
- Strong Ale
- Sour Ale
- Wheat Beer
- Zwickelbier

• • • • • • • • •

Major Planets of our Solar System (8)

- Mercury
- Venus
- Earth
- Mars
- Jupiter
- Saturn
- Uranus
- Neptune

LIST 15

• • • • • • • • •

Ivy League Universities (8)

- Brown University
- Columbia University
- Cornell University
- Dartmouth College
- Harvard University
- University of Pennsylvania
- Princeton University
- Yale University

Possible Blood Types (8)

- O Negative
- O Positive
- A Negative
- A Positive
- B Negative
- B Positive
- AB Negative
- AB Positive

● ● ● ● ● ● ● ● ●

Main Hawaiian Islands (8)

- Hawai'i - The Big Island
- Maui - The Valley Isle
- O'ahu - The Gathering Place
- Kaua'i - The Garden Isle
- Moloka'i - The Friendly Isle
- Lana'i - The Pineapple Isle
- Ni'ihau - The Forbidden Isle
- Kaho'olawe - The Target Isle

List 18

Muhammed Ali Legacy Award Recipients 2014 - 2020 (9)

- Magic Johnson - 2014
- Jack Nicklaus - 2015
- Jim Brown - 2016
- Bill Russell - 2016
- Kareem Abdul-Jabbar - 2016
- Colin Kaepernick - 2017
- John Cena - 2018
- Warrick Dunn - 2019
- LeBron James - 2020

● ● ● ● ● ● ● ● ●

Santa's Reindeers (9)

- Dasher
- Dancer
- Prancer
- Vixen
- Comet
- Cupid
- Donner
- Blitzen
- Rudolph

LIST 20

Current Supreme Court Justices (9)

- John G. Roberts, Jr. - Chief Justice of the United States
- Clarence Thomas - Associate Justice
- Stephen G. Breyer - Associate Justice
- Samuel A. Alito, Jr. - Associate Justice
- Sonia Sotomayor - Associate Justice
- Elena Kagan - Associate Justice
- Neil M. Gorsuch - Associate Justice
- Brett M. Kavanaugh - Associate Justice
- Amy Coney Barrett - Associate Justice

● ● ● ● ● ● ● ● ●

McDonald's 1948 Original Menu (9)

- Hamburgers
- Cheese Burgers
- Fries
- Milk
- Root Beer
- Orangeade
- Coca Cola
- Coffee
- Milkshakes (chocolate, vanilla, strawberry)

● ● ● ● ● ● ● ● ●

Oldest Video Games in the World (1st 10)

- Gun Fight - 1975
- Tank - 1974
- Gran Trak 10 - 1974
- Space Race - 1973
- Pong - 1972
- Magnavox Odyssey Games - 1972
- Galaxy Game - 1971
- Computer Space - 1971
- Space War 1 - 1962
- Tennis for Two - 1958

Oldest Hotels in Las Vegas (1st 10)

- Holiday Casino - 1973
- Circus Circus - 1968
- Caesars Palace - 1966
- Flamingo Capri - 1959
- Tropicana - 1957
- Sahara Hotel & Casino - 1952
- Flamingo Hotel & Casino - 1946
- The Golden Nugget Saloon - 1946
- El Cortez - 1941
- Hotel Nevada - 1906

Major Body Organs (10)

- Brain
- Lungs
- Liver
- Bladder
- Kidneys
- Stomach
- Heart
- Intestines
- Muscles
- Skin

Tea Producing Countries (Top 10)

- China
- India
- Kenya
- Sri Lanka
- Turkey
- Indonesia
- Vietnam
- Japan
- Iran
- Argentina

● ● ● ● ● ● ● ● ●

Rodgers and Hammerstein Musicals (11)

- Oklahoma - 1943
- Carousel - 1945
- Allegro - 1947
- South Pacific - 1949
- The King and I - 1951
- Me and Juliet - 1953
- Pipe Dream - 1955
- Flower Drum Song - 1958
- The Sound of Music - 1959
- State Fair - 1996
- Cinderella - 2013

Color Theory
(12 + Black & White)

Primary Colors (3)
- Red
- Yellow
- Blue

Secondary Colors (3)
- Orange (mixture of Red & Yellow)
- Green (mixture of Yellow & Blue)
- Purple (mixture of Blue & Red)

Black and White (2)

Primary Colors of Light (3)
- Red
- Green
- Blue

Complementary Colors of Light (3)
- Yellow (complement of Blue)
- Cyan (complement of Red)
- Magenta (complement of Green)

Astronauts Who Have Stepped on the Moon (12)

- Neil Armstrong
- Buzz Aldrin
- Pete Conrad
- Alan Bean
- Alan Shepard
- Edgar Mitchell
- David Scott
- James Irwin
- John Young
- Charles Duke
- Eugene Cernan
- Harrison Schmitt

The Apostles (12)

- Peter
- Andrew
- James
- John
- Phillip
- Bartholomew
- Thomas
- Matthew
- James (son of Alphaeus)
- Thaddaeus
- Simon
- Judas Iscariot (replaced by Matthias)

Chinese Zodiac Animal Signs (12)

- Rat
- Ox
- Tiger
- Rabbit
- Dragon
- Snake
- Horse
- Sheep
- Monkey
- Rooster
- Dog
- Pig

LIST 31

●●●●●●●●●

Canadian Provinces and Territories (13)

- Nunavut
- Quebec
- Northwest Territories
- Ontario
- British Columbia
- Alberta
- Saskatchewan
- Manitoba
- Yukon
- Newfoundland and Labrador
- New Brunswick
- Nova Scotia
- Prince Edward Island

Greek Mythology's Mt. Olympus Gods & Goddesses (13)

- Hades
- Zeus
- Poseidon
- Apollo
- Ares
- Dionysus
- Hephaestus
- Hestia
- Demeter
- Hera
- Artemis
- Athena
- Aphrodite

• • • • • • • • •

Quarterbacks to Throw 99yd TD Passes (13)

- Frank Filchock - 1939
- George Izo - 1963
- Karl Sweetan - 1966
- Sonny Jurgensen - 1966
- Jim Plunkett - 1983
- Ron Jaworski - 1985
- Stan Humphries - 1985
- Brett Favre - 1995
- Trent Green - 2002
- Jeff Garcia - 2004
- Gus Frerotte - 2008
- Tom Brady - 2008
- Eli Manning - 2011

America's Original Colonies (13)

- Virginia
- Massachusetts
- New Hampshire
- Maryland
- Connecticut
- Rhode Island & Providence Plantations
- Delaware
- North Carolina
- South Carolina
- New Jersey
- New York
- Pennsylvania
- Georgia

Cloud Types (14)

High Clouds (3)
- Cirrus
- Cirrostratus
- Cirrocumulus

Mid-level Clouds (3)
- Altocumulus
- Altostratus
- Nimbostratus

Low Clouds (4)
- Cumulus
- Stratus
- Cumulonimbus
- Stratocumulus

Special Clouds (4)
- Contrails
- Mammatus
- Orographic
- Lenticular

U. S. Territories (14)

- American Samoa
- Baker Island
- Guam
- Howland Island
- Jarvis Island
- Johnston Atoll
- Kingman Reef
- Midway Islands
- Navassa Island
- Northern Mariana Islands
- Palmyra Atoll
- Puerto Rico
- U. S. Virgin Islands
- Wake Islands

Original Looney Tunes Characters (15)

- Bugs Bunny
- Daffy Duck
- Porky Pig
- Elmer Fudd
- Wile E. Coyote
- Road Runner
- Speedy Gonzales
- Yosemite Sam
- Tasmanian Devil
- Marvin the Martian
- Foghorn Leghorn
- Pepe' Le Pew
- Sylvester the Cat
- Tweety Bird
- Granny

Most Popular Edible Mushrooms (15)

- Hedgehog
- Portobello
- Button
- Shitake
- Wood Blewit
- Matsutake
- Lion's Mane
- Reishi
- Maitake
- Oyster
- Cremini
- Morel
- Porcini
- Enoki
- Chanterelle

LIST 39

● ● ● ● ● ● ● ● ●

Star Wars Movie Series in Chronological Order (16)

- Star Wars: Episode I -The Phantom Menace
- Star Wars: Episode II - Attack of the Clones
- Star Wars: The Clone Wars
- Solo: A Star Wars Story
- Star Wars: Episode III - Revenge of the Sith
- Star Wars: Revelations
- Rogue One: A Star Wars Story
- Star Wars: Episode IV - A New Hope
- The Star Wars Holiday Special
- Star Wars: Episode V - The Empire Strikes Back
- Ewoks: The Battle for Endor
- The Ewok Adventure
- Star Wars: Episode VI - Return of the Jedi
- Star Wars: Episode VII - The Force Awakens
- Star Wars: Episode VIII - The Last Jedi
- Star Wars: Episode IX - The Rise of Skywalker

Boxing Weight Classes (17)

- Heavyweight - Unlimited
- Cruiserweight - 200 lbs.
- Light heavyweight - 175 lbs.
- Super middleweight - 168 lbs.
- Middleweight - 160 lbs.
- Junior middleweight - 154 lbs.
- Welterweight - 147 lbs.
- Junior welterweight - 140 lbs.
- Lightweight - 135 lbs.
- Junior lightweight - 130 lbs.
- Featherweight - 126 lbs
- Junior featherweight - 122 lbs.
- Bantamweight - 118 lbs.
- Junior bantamweight - 115 lbs.
- Flyweight - 112 lbs.
- Jr. flyweight - 108 lbs.
- Strawweight - 105 lbs

"Peanuts" Comic Strip Characters (18)

- Charlie Brown
- Patty - Early character
- Shermy
- Snoopy
- Violet Gray
- Schroeder
- Lucy Van Pelt
- Linus Van Pelt
- Pig Pen
- Sally Brown
- Frieda
- Woodstock
- Peppermint Patty
- Franklin
- Marcie
- Rerun Van Pelt
- Eudora
- Peggy Jean

Major *Seas* of the World (18)

- Baffin Bay
- Labrador Sea
- Hudson Bay
- Gulf of Mexico
- Caribbean Sea
- Greenland Sea
- Norwegian Sea
- North Sea
- Mediterranean Sea
- Black Sea
- Caspian Sea
- Red Sea
- Persian Gulf
- Arabian Sea
- Bay of Bengal
- South China Sea
- East China Sea
- Sea of Japan

Metric System Prefixes and Units (19)

- Exa
- Peta
- Tera
- Giga
- Mega
- Kilo
- Hecto
- Deka
- **Meter - Unit = 1**
- **Gram - Unit =1**
- **Liter - Unit = 1**
- Deci
- Centi
- Milli
- Micro
- Nano
- Pico
- Femto
- Atto

* Prefixes above the units = more than the unit
* Prefixes below the units = less than the unit

List 44

•••••••••

Faces on
U. S. Currency (20)

Coin
- President Abraham Lincoln - Penny
- President Thomas Jefferson - Nickel
- President Franklin D. Roosevelt - Dime
- President George Washington - Quarter
- President John F. Kennedy - Half Dollar
- Lady Liberty - $1 Dollar
- 1st Woman to Vote, Susan B. Anthony - $1 Dollar
- Explorer Sacagawea - $1 Dollar

Paper Bills
- President George Washington - $1 Dollar
- President Thomas Jefferson - $2 Dollar
- President Abraham Lincoln - $5 Dollar
- Alexander Hamilton - $10 Dollar
- President Andrew Jackson - $20 Dollar
- President Ulysses S. Grant - $50 Dollar
- Benjamin Franklin - $100 Dollar
- President William McKinley - $500 Dollar
- President Grover Cleveland - $1,000 Dollar
- President James Madison - $5,000 Dollar
- Salmon P. Chase - $10,000 Dollar
- President Woodrow Wilson - $100,000 Dollar

LIST 45

• • • • • • • • •

Executive Cabinet Positions (21)

- Secretary of State
- Secretary of the Treasury
- Secretary of Defense
- Attorney General
- Secretary of the Interior
- Secretary of Agriculture
- Secretary of Commerce
- Secretary of Labor
- Secretary of Health and Human Services
- Secretary of Housing and Urban Development
- Secretary of Transportation
- Secretary of Energy
- Secretary of Education
- Secretary of Veterans Affairs
- Secretary of Homeland Security
- Trade Representative
- Director of National Intelligence
- Director of the Office of Management and Budget
- Director of the Central Intelligence Agency
- Administrator of the Environmental Protection Agency
- Administrator of the Small Business Administration

● ● ● ● ● ● ● ● ●

Olympic Hosts - Countries (23)

- Austria - Winter
- Australia - Summer
- Belgium - Summer
- Brazil - Summer
- Canada - Summer/Winter
- China - Summer/Winter*
- Finland - Summer
- France - Summer/Winter
- Germany - Summer/Winter
- Greece - Summer
- Italy - Summer/Winter
- Japan - Summer/Winter
- Mexico - Summer
- Netherlands - Summer
- Norway - Winter
- Russia - Summer/Winter
- Spain - Summer
- South Korea - Summer/Winter
- Sweden - Summer
- Switzerland - Winter
- United Kingdom - Summer
- United States - Summer/Winter
- Yugoslavia - Winter

● ● ● ● ● ● ● ● ●

Greek Alphabet (24)

- Alpha
- Beta
- Gamma
- Delta
- Epsilon
- Zeta
- Eta
- Theta
- Iota
- Kappa
- Lambda
- Mu

- Nu
- Xi
- Omicron
- Pi
- Rho
- Sigma
- Tau
- Upsilon
- Phi
- Chi
- Psi
- Omega

Prime Numbers Between 1-100 (25)

- 2
- 3
- 5
- 7
- 11
- 13
- 17
- 19
- 23
- 29
- 31
- 37
- 41
- 43
- 47
- 53
- 59
- 61
- 67
- 71
- 73
- 79
- 83
- 89
- 97

Phonetic Alphabet (26)

- Alpha
- Bravo
- Charlie
- Delta
- Echo
- Foxtrot
- Golf
- Hotel
- India
- Juliet
- Kilo
- Lima
- Mike

- November
- Oscar
- Papa
- Quebec
- Romeo
- Sierra
- Tango
- Uniform
- Victor
- Whiskey
- X-ray
- Yankee
- Zulu

• • • • • • • • •

North American Hummingbirds (27)

- Allen's
- Amethyst-throated
- Anna's
- Antillean Crested
- Bahama Woodstar
- Bee
- Berylline
- Black Chinned
- Blue-throated
- Broad-billed
- Broad-tailed
- Buff-bellied
- Bumblebee
- Calliope
- Cinnamon
- Costa's
- Cuban Emerald
- Green-breasted Mango
- Lucifer
- Mexican Violetear
- Plain-capped Starthroat
- Rivoli's
- Ruby-throated
- Rufous
- Velvet-crowned
- White-eared
- Xantus's

Major League Baseball 500 Home Run Club (27)

- Barry Bonds
- Hank Aaron
- Babe Ruth
- Alex Rodriguez
- Willie Mays
- Ken Griffey Jr.
- Albert Pujols
- Jim Thome
- Sammy Sosa
- Frank Robinson
- Mark McGwire
- Harmon Killebrew
- Rafael Palmeiro
- Reggie Jackson
- Manny Ramirez
- Mike Schmidt
- David Ortiz
- Mickey Mantle
- Jimmie Foxx
- Willie McCovey
- Frank Thomas
- Ted Williams
- Ernie Banks
- Eddie Matthews
- Mel Ott
- Gary Sheffield
- Eddie Murray

Monopoly Game Properties (28)

- Atlantic Avenue
- B & O Railroad
- Baltic Avenue
- Boardwalk
- Connecticut Avenue
- Electric Company
- Illinois Avenue
- Indiana Avenue
- Kentucky Avenue
- Marvin Gardens
- Mediterranean Avenue
- New York Avenue
- North Carolina Avenue
- Oriental Avenue
- Pacific Avenue
- Park Place
- Pennsylvania Avenue
- Pennsylvania Railroad
- Reading Railroad
- Short Line
- St. Charles Place
- St. James Place
- States Avenue
- Tennessee Avenue
- Ventnor Avenue
- Vermont Avenue
- Virginia Avenue
- Water Works

● ● ● ● ● ● ● ● ●

Women's Singles Champions Having 5 & More Tennis Grand Slam Titles (30)

- Margaret Court - 24
- Serena Williams - 23
- Steffi Graff - 22
- Helen Wills Moody - 19
- Chris Evert - 18
- Martina Navratilova - 18
- Billie Jean King - 12
- Maureen Connolly - 9
- Monica Seles - 9
- Suzanne Lenglen - 8
- Molla Bjurstedt Mallory - 8
- Dorothea Lambert Chambers - 7
- Maria Bueno - 7
- Evonne Goolagong - 7
- Justine Henin - 7
- Venus Williams - 7
- Blanche Bingley Hillyard - 6
- Margaret Osborne - 6
- Nancye Wynne Bolton - 6
- Louise Brough - 6
- Doris Hart - 6
- Lottie Dod - 5
- Charlotte Cooper Sterry - 5
- Daphne Akhurst - 5
- Helen Jacobs - 5
- Alice Marble - 5
- Pauline Betz - 5
- Althea Gibson - 5
- Martina Hingis - 5
- Maria Sharapova - 5

States of Mexico (31)

- Aguascalientes
- Baja California
- Baja California Sur
- Campeche
- Chiapas
- *Mexico City
- Chihuahua
- Coahuila
- Colima
- Durango
- Guanajuato
- Guerrero
- Hidalgo
- Jalisco
- Mexico
- Michoacan

- Morelos
- Nayarit
- Nuevo Leon
- Oaxaca
- Puebla
- Queretaro
- Quintana Roo
- San Luis Potosi
- Sinaloa
- Sonora
- Tabasco
- Tamaulipas
- Tlaxcala
- Veracruz
- Yucatan
- Zacatecas

Performers at Woodstock Music and Arts Festival (33)

- Richie Havens
- Swami Satchidananda
- Sweetwater
- Bert Sommer
- Tim Harden
- Ravi Shankar
- Melanie
- Arlo Guthrie
- Joan Baez
- Quill
- Country Joe McDonald
- Santana
- John Sebastian
- Keef Hartley Band
- The Incredible String Band
- Canned Heat
- Mountain
- Grateful Dead
- Creedence Clearwater Revival
- Janis Joplin and the Kozmic Blues Band
- Sly & the Family Stone
- The Who
- Jefferson Airplane
- Joe Cocker and the Grease Band
- Country Joe and the Fish
- Ten Years After
- The Band
- Johnny Winter
- Blood Sweat & Tears
- Crosby, Stills, Nash & Young
- Paul Butterfield Blues Band
- Sha Na Na
- Jimi Hendrix

Transition Metals (38)

- Scandium
- Titanium
- Vanadium
- Chromium
- Manganese
- Iron
- Cobalt
- Nickel
- Copper
- Zinc
- Yttrium
- Zirconium
- Niobium
- Molybdenum
- Technetium
- Ruthenium
- Rhodium
- Palladium
- Silver
- Cadmium
- Hafnium
- Tantalum
- Tungsten
- Rhenium
- Osmium
- Iridium
- Platinum
- Gold
- Mercury
- Rutherfordium
- Dubnium
- Seaborgium
- Bohrium
- Hassium
- Meitnerium
- Ununnilium
- Unununium
- Ununbium

CBS "60 Minutes" Hosts, Correspondents, & Commentators (51)

Current Hosts

- Leslie Stahl
- Scott Pelley
- Bill Whitaker
- John Dickerson

Former Hosts

- Harry Reasoner
- Mike Wallace
- Morley Safer
- Dan Rather
- Ed Bradley
- Diane Sawyer
- Meredith Vieira
- Bob Simon
- Christiane Amanpour
- Lara Logan
- Steve Kroft

Current Part-Time Correspondents

- Anderson Cooper
- Norah O'Donnell
- Sharyn Alfonsi
- Jon Wertheim

Former Part-Time Correspondents

- Walter Cronkite
- Charles Kuralt
- Roger Mudd
- Bill Plante
- Eric Sevareid
- John Hart
- Bob Schieffer
- Morton Dean
- Marlene Sanders
- Charles Osgood
- Forrest Sawyer
- Connie Chung
- Paula Zahn
- John Roberts
- Russ Mitchell
- Carol Marin
- Bryant Gumbel
- Katie Couric
- Charlie Rose
- Byron Pitts
- Alison Stewart
- Sanjay Gupta
- Oprah Winfrey

Commentators

- James J. Kilpatrick
- Nicholas von Hoffman
- Shana Alexander
- Andy Rooney
- Stanley Crouch
- Molly Ivins
- P. J. O'Rourke
- Bill Clinton
- Bob Dole

Crayola's Crayon Colors (Box of 64)

- Apricot
- Asparagus
- Bittersweet
- Black
- Blue
- Blue Green
- Blue Violet
- Brick
- Brown
- Burnt Orange
- Burnt Sienna
- Cadet Blue
- Cerulean
- Chestnut
- Cornflower
- Dandelion
- Forest Green
- Gold
- Goldenrod
- Grammy Smith Apple
- Gray
- Green
- Green Yellow
- Indigo
- Lavender
- Macaroni and Cheese
- Magenta
- Mahogany
- Mauvelous
- Melon
- Orange
- Orchid
- Olive Green
- Pacific Blue
- Peach
- Periwinkle
- Pink Carnation
- Plum
- Potter's Orange

- Purple Mountain's Majesty
- Raw Sienna
- Red
- Red Orange
- Red Violet
- Robin's Egg Blue
- Salmon
- Scarlet
- Sea Green
- Sepia
- Silver
- Sky Blue
- Spring Green
- Tan
- Tickle Me Pink
- Timberwolf
- Tumbleweed
- Turquoise
- Violet
- Violet Red
- White
- Wild Strawberry
- Wisteria
- Yellow
- Yellow Orange

Current Countries Having Participated in "FIFA" World Cup Soccer (86)

- Albania
- Algeria
- Angola
- Antigua & Barbuda
- Argentina
- Australia
- Austria
- Belgium
- Bhutan
- Bolivia
- Bosnia & Herzegovina
- Brazil
- Bulgaria
- Cameroon
- Canada
- Chile
- China
- Colombia
- Costa Rica
- Cote d'Ivoire
- Croatia
- Cuba
- Czech Republic
- Denmark
- Ecuador
- Egypt
- El Salvador
- England
- Estonia
- France
- Germany
- Ghana
- Greece
- Haiti
- Honduras

- Hungary
- Iceland
- India
- Indonesia
- Iran
- Iraq
- Ireland
- Israel
- Italy
- Japan
- Kuwait
- Luxembourg
- Mexico
- Montserrat
- Morocco
- Netherlands
- New Zealand
- Nigeria
- Northern Ireland
- North Korea
- Norway
- Panama
- Paraguay
- Peru
- Poland
- Portugal
- Romania
- Russia
- Saudi Arabia
- Scotland
- Senegal
- Serbia
- Slovakia
- Slovenia
- Sri Lanka
- South Africa
- South Korea
- Spain
- Sudan
- Sweden
- Switzerland
- Toga
- Trinidad & Tobago
- Tunisia
- Turkey
- Ukraine
- Uruguay
- USA
- Wales
- Zaire
- Zambia

● ● ● ● ● ● ● ● ●

Officially Recognized Constellations (88)

- Andromeda
- Antlia
- Apus
- Aquarius
- Aquila
- Ara
- Aries
- Auriga
- Bootes
- Caelum
- Camelopardalis
- Cancer
- Canes Venatici
- Canis Major
- Canis Minor
- Capricornus
- Carina
- Cassiopeia
- Centaurus
- Cepheus
- Cetus
- Chamaeleon
- Circinus
- Columba
- Coma Berenices
- Corona Australis
- Corona Borealis
- Corvus
- Crater
- Crux
- Cygnus
- Delphinus
- Dorado
- Draco
- Equuleus
- Eridanus
- Fornax
- Gemini
- Grus
- Hercules
- Horologium
- Hydra

- Hydrus
- Indus
- Lacerta
- Leo
- Leo Minor
- Lepus
- Libra
- Lupus
- Lynx
- Lyra
- Mensa
- Microscopium
- Monoceros
- Musca
- Norma
- Octans
- Ophiuchus
- Orion
- Pavo
- Pegasus
- Perseus
- Phoenix
- Pictor
- Pisces
- Piscis Austrinus
- Puppis
- Pyxis
- Reticulum
- Sagitta
- Sagittarius
- Scorpius
- Sculptor
- Scutum
- Serpens
- Sextans
- Taurus
- Telescopium
- Triangulum
- Triangulum Australe
- Tucana
- Ursa Major
- Ursa Minor
- Vela
- Virgo
- Volans
- Vulpecula

CPSIA information can be obtained
at www.ICGtesting.com
Printed in the USA
LVHW022158080222
710545LV00009B/471